The Beverly Hillbillies Diet

Glenda Ruby

The Beverly Hillbillies Diet

Welcome to the World of the Golden Grit!

BEAUFORT BOOKS, INC.

New York/Toronto

Line drawings on pages 12, 22, 24, 26, 28, 30, 34, 36, 68, and 70 reprinted
courtesy of The New York Public Library.

Library of Congress Cataloging in Publication Data

Ruby, Glenda.
  The Beverly Hillbillies diet.

  1. Reducing diets—Recipes. I. Title.
RM222.2.R84   1982   613.2′5   82-4328
ISBN 0-8253-0100-9 (pbk.)   AACR2

Published in the United States by Beaufort Books, Inc., New York. Published simultaneously in Canada by General Publishing Co. Limited

Designer: Ellen LoGiudice

Printed in the U.S.A.   First Edition
    10 9 8 7 6 5 4 3 2 1

Acknowledgements

I would like to acknowledge the great assistance of Betty Ruby, a Quadruple Grand Champion of The Blowing Springs Bake-Off and my dear mother; and that of Missy McMillan, a five-time winner of the Pan-Mississippi Confection Contest; and her daughter, my friend, Suzanne, for their kindness in sharing heirloom recipes with all of us.

Both my parents, Betty and George, have my deepest appreciation for their constant encouragement and shipments of pickles and pot holders.

For their very generous support, I especially want to say how grateful I am to Candace Gimber and Spats.

I certainly want to thank my southern sisters, clever Rowena Upham Brown (and her husband Robinson, a grit by marriage), and the vivacious Ann Cunningham for their enthusiasm and guidance. Also thanks to my southern brother, Arthur Lavidge III, for his floured board flourishes.

I want to give Lifetime Grit Gift Certificates to Michael West, Viena Margulies, and Ray Winship who fed me faithfully when I couldn't face another frying pan.

This book is better for the wit of the editor, Susan Suffes, and for her patience and impatience. And better for the help of our designer, Ellen LoGiudice.

Also, thanks and a pan of corn bread to Eric Kampmann, for his uncommon good sense in taking me as a client.

And, finally, thanks to Paul Henning and Norman Tyre for their cooperation in extending permission to use the name of Paul's very funny show, "The Beverly Hillbillies," without which there would have been no title and no book.

Contents

1
Welcome to the World of the Golden Grit

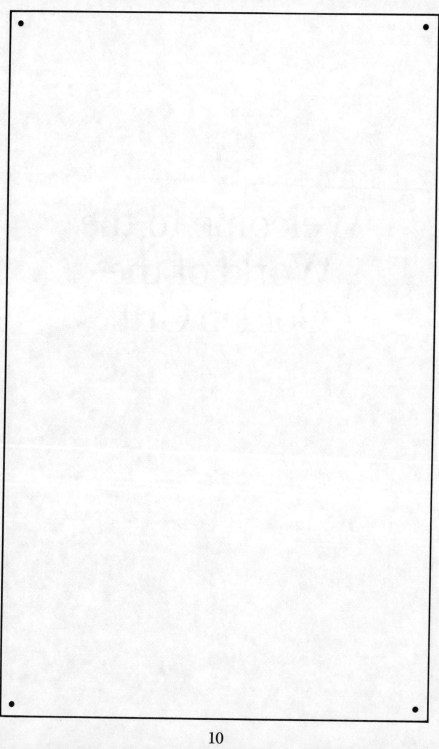

You may be among thousands of city folks who waddle into their bathrooms one morning, clamber up on their scales, and find they have become bigger than they have any business being.

In some cases, big enough to go bear hunting with a switch.

Many of these folks have accidentally become fat because their eating habits have become *citified.* Take this simple quiz and ask yourself:

- Do *you* require *two* seats at screenings?

- Have Budweiser or Earl Scheib tried to rent your back for advertising?

- Can you recite the menu at Ma Maison?

- Does your crossing the street cause gridlock?

- Could you wear Orson Welles's hand-me-downs?

- When you come to a fork in the road, do you reach for it?

Inside every fat city person there's a fit hillbilly trying to get back to the basics.

Haven't you climbed into your crinoline and exclaimed, "Mercy! There's so much of me!"

Or gone to button your suit . . . in vain?

The Beverly Hillbillies Diet can help you all out in several ways:

First: It will help you shape up.

Second: It will help you break the dependence you have on city foods.

Third: It will help you bring the good old days back to your table.

Some diets ask you to weigh your food. This is nothing but foolishness because it's *you* on a diet, not your food.

Other diets tell you to eat only exotic fruits. These diets can have unusual side effects, mainly an odd tendency to break into a hula at the sight of a supermarket. A pear is no substitute for a porkchop.

We believe that if you keep in touch with the land you will also be able to touch your toes. Keep in mind that most of us, as our dear friend Johnny Carson points out, are country people at heart.

Just because somewhere along the line you got off track and your waistline got away from you doesn't mean you can't get back to the basics and be fit as a fiddle.

The good old days

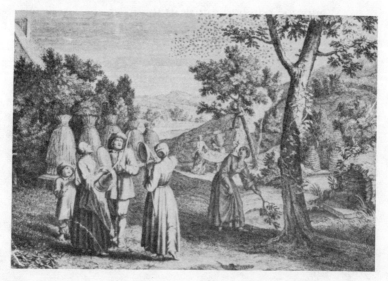

2
How City Folks Get Fat

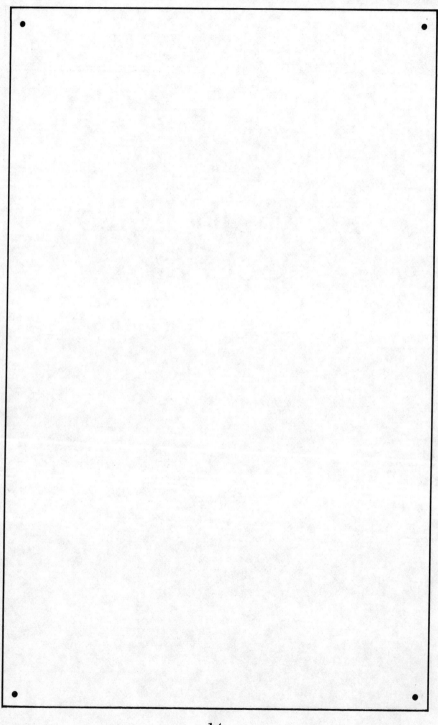

HOW CITY FOLKS GET FAT

1. **They never walk anywhere.**

   FACK*: You gain a pound for every five miles you ride when you could have walked. *The Beverly Hillbillies Diet* will put your little old feet right back on the ground.

2. **They eat too much foreign food.**

   FACK: Foreign food will make you gain weight; look at anybody named Pierre or Luciano. On *The Beverly Hillbillies Diet,* you will eat down-home-style food, not alien eats. We are going to help you return to cast-iron cuisine while leading you down your own garden path.

3. **Too much is done for them.**

   FACK: Keep a garden and your garden will keep you. When you stray from the country life, you will find your clothes commence to strain at the seams. And, if you had to *grow* most of the things you eat, you would surely lose weight, at least until the radishes come up.

---

* That's right, fack (that's "fact" to anyone who has never been south of Bloomingdale's).

THE FOUR TYPES OF CITY FAT

1. **Polite Fat.**

   City folks tend to do business while sitting down to lunch or dinner. Some of you feel that holding up your end of the conversation also means holding up your fork.

   This is how so many city folks get too big for their britches.

2. **Nervous Fat.**

   The minute city folks get bugged about something, they try to calm down by chowing down. A frantic trip to the feeding trough may temporarily settle your nerves, but the food also settles permanently on the old bottom.

   Unfortunately, digestion is not the best cure for agitation.

3. **Sad Fat.**

   There are folks who try to banish the mopes with a nice helping of Veal Milanese forgetting how sad they will be later standing on the scales.

   You cannot beat the blues with Baked Alaska.

4. **Fast Fat.**

   Hectic city schedules don't always leave much time to eat, so like as not a city person will run into a fast food place for a quick quart of french fries and a bogusburger.

   Counting these calories is about as easy as counting confetti.

CITY FAT MYTHS

City folks—who should know better—are suckered into believing that:

- You have to eat to be popular.

- Three meals a day keep the doctor away.

- Snips and snails and lobster tails—that's what little boys are made of.

- Men seldom make glaces for girls who wear glasses.

- The best things in life are sugar-free.

- Every torte has a heart of gold.

These examples of gross misinformation soon develop into the dreaded signs of compulsive city eating.

SIGNS OF COMPULSIVE CITY EATING

- Eating a Sabrett's with the napkin still around it.

- Buying burritos by the six-pack.

- Eating pizza at a baseball game (it can't be much good; baseball isn't even played in Italy).

- A brass plaque on your table at L'Ermitage.

- Charge accounts at Chock Full O' Nuts and Häagen-Dazs.

- Only reserving limos with radar ranges.

- Flecks of bearnaise in your toupee.

- A Julia Child tattoo.

- Bagel earrings.

- A Cuisinart in your glove compartment.

Don't despair; all is not lost. The only thing you have to lose is half a ton.

But, you say, I just want to be svelte . . . I don't want to starve.

You won't starve—*if* you follow *The Beverly Hillbillies Diet* Food Groups and Weekly Diet Plans.

3

The Beverly Hillbillies Diet Food Groups

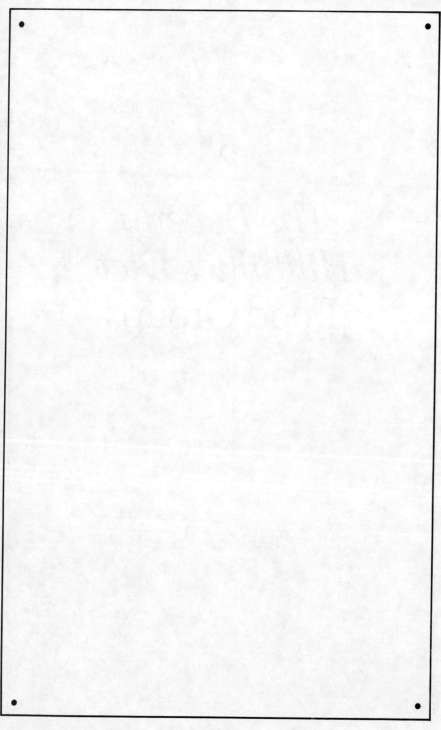

1. THE PIG

Barbecue • Ham • Fatback • Sausage • Bacon • Porkchops • Pork Roast

2. THE POND

Catfish • Crappie • Frog legs • Bream • Trout • Bass • Crawfish

3. THE PATCH AND THE ORCHARD

Mustard greens • Okra • Peppers • Radishes • Collard greens • Squash • Carrots • Polk salad • Tomatoes • Beans • Corn • Onions • Potatoes • Peas • Herbs • Garlic • Cucumbers • Melons • Grapes • Leeks.
Apple, plum, cherry, pear, hickory, walnut, and pecan trees

4. THE HENHOUSE AND OLD BOSSY

Eggs • Milk • Cheese • Butter • Cream • Chicken • Sour cream • Buttermilk

5. THE BREAD BOX

Biscuits • Hushpuppies • Spoon bread • Corn bread • Griddle cakes • Banana bread • Grits

6. THE PANTRY

Green tomato pickles • Preserves, jams, jellies • Bread and butter pickles • Chow-chow

7. STORE-BOUGHT

Caviar • Condiments.
Champagne, port, whiskey, wines • Brie

8. JUST DESSERTS

Banana pudding • Chess pie • Pecan pie • Divinity • Peach cobbler • Sweet potato pie • Pineapple upside-down cake

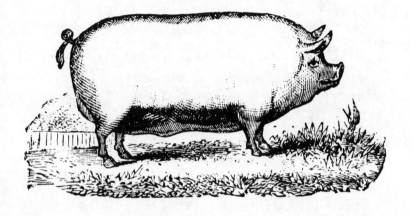

The pig

Now let's break these vittles down one step more.

1. THE PIG

Barbecue • Ham • Fatback • Sausage • Bacon • Porkchops • Pork roast

As you can see from the delicious array of eats, The Pig is a serviceable beast and might near a complete life-support system all by itself. Apart from providing these delectable morsels, the Pig Group can mean a lot of hustle for your bustle, say:

Activity	Calories burned
Addressing invitations	1500
Digging a barbecue pit	5000
Splitting wood for a barbecue	700
Carrying cases of beer and ice, and washtubs to the barbecue area	200
Setting up hammocks and yard furniture	150
Turning the spit off and on all day	375

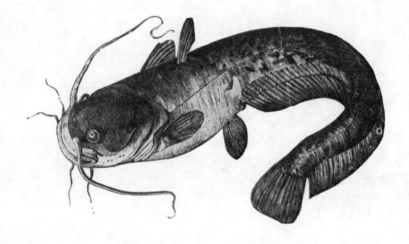

The catfish

2. THE POND

Catfish • Crappie • Frog legs • Bream • Trout • Bass • Crawfish

On your way to catching and enjoying the palatable pleasures of The Pond, you will also enjoy wonderfully improved muscle tone, as you

Activity	Calories burned
Leap around half an hour catching grasshoppers for bait	240
Squat for an hour digging worms and grubs	190
Clamber about a mile through briars and across cow pastures, hauling bait, tackle, and lunch bucket, to the pond	275
Cast and reel all day, then clean the fish	535
Discuss your fishing trip after dinner	300

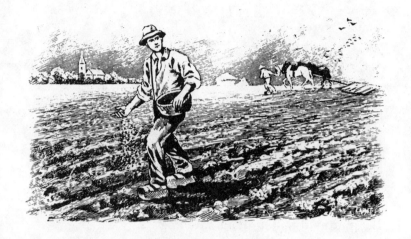

The patch and the orchard

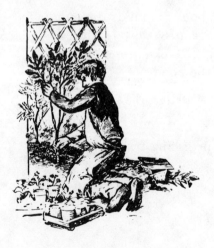

3. THE PATCH AND THE ORCHARD

Collard greens • Okra • Peppers • Radishes • Mustard greens • Squash • Carrots • Polk salad • Tomatoes • Beans • Corn • Onions • Potatoes • Peas • Herbs • Garlic • Cucumbers • Melons • Grapes • Leeks
Apple, plum, cherry, pear, hickory, walnut, and pecan trees

Since you can't eat it until you've grown it, The Patch offers a passle of opportunities to lose weight.

Lots of former fatties say that putting in their very own vegetable patch was the best thing about *The Beverly Hillbillies Diet*, next to eating fried okra, fried corn, and fried tomatoes.

And it suited their waistlines just fine!

Activity	Calories burned
Decide where the garden should be (four-hour conversation)	300
Purchase tools, seeds, shoots	90
Put in garden	4,750,000
Build in scarecrow	1200
Weed and water as necessary	225
Pick potato bugs	125
Pick a peck of peppers	375

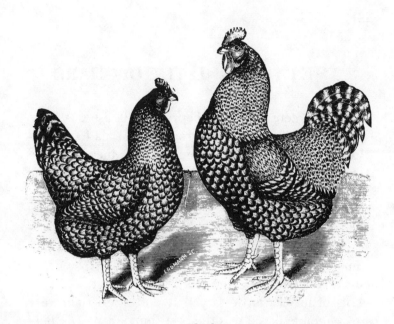

The hen

Old bossy

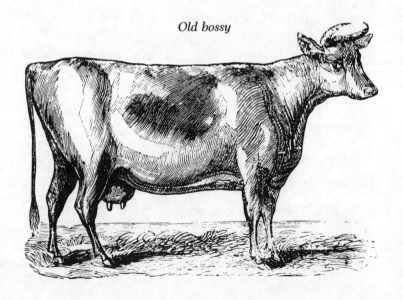

4. THE HENHOUSE AND OLD BOSSY

Eggs • Milk • Cheese • Butter • Cream • Chicken • Sour cream • Buttermilk

There are some great opportunities here to get to know these animals and make them your friends. After all, they do make your breakfasts, lunches, and dinners.

Activity	Calories burned
Hauling chicken feed	350
Pitching hay for Old Bossy	575
Milking Old Bossy	150
Interviewing hired hand to pitch hay and milk old Bossy and haul chicken feed	325
Catching a fryer for dinner	200
Searching antique stores for churn	550

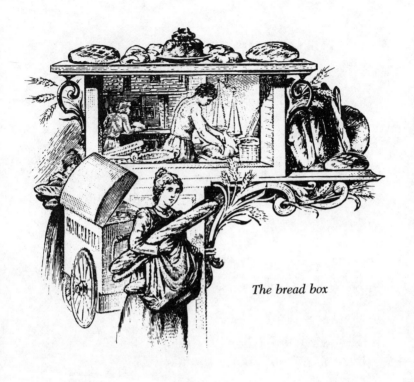

The bread box

5. THE BREAD BOX

Biscuits • Hushpuppies • Spoon bread • Corn bread •
Griddle cakes • Banana bread • Grits

Learning to make good biscuits will not only tone the
muscles in your arms, it will build character. Corn bread
is one of the staples of a solid, basic diet and is a country
texture you can combine with all the other food groups.

Activity	Calories burned
Looking for lard	10,000
Breaking in your rolling pin	230
Kneading all you need to	350
Self-control enough not to inhale rolls or cornbread the minute they come out of the oven	75
Passing the biscuits	25 per pass

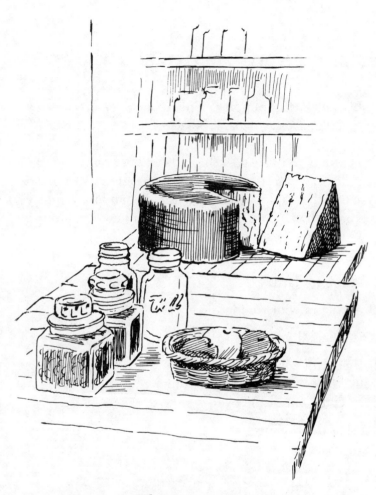

The pantry

6. THE PANTRY

Green tomato pickles • Preserves, jams, jellies • Bread and butter pickles • Chow-chow

Once you get cracking on this section of *The Beverly Hillbillies Diet*, you won't have much time to eat; for a while you'll be too busy to take nary a mouthful.

But a little later on, you'll have one fine time; you'll have some fine compliments from the family and some fine complements to the other food groups.

Activity	Calories burned
Carry jars home from the store	350
Pick a peck of peppers ... and to-matoes and cucumbers	245
Slice, dice, grind, peel, core, chop, cut, strain, and so on	430
Walk up and down step ladder 40 or 50 times placing jars on shelf one at a time	325
Design label for jars, e.g., "Trellis Mae's Put-Up Treasures"	100
Hand-deliver samples to neighbors, relatives, and shut-ins	580

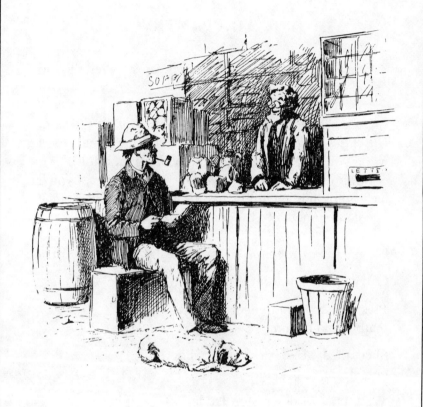

The store

7. STORE-BOUGHT

Caviar • Condiments • Champagne, whiskey, port, wines • Brie

Buy anything you like and eat hearty, but remember: You have to walk to and from the store toting the groceries.

Activity	Calories burned
Pushing buggy with one bum wheel	135
Going up and down each aisle at least once	165
Negotiating case price for wine	215
Hefting magnum ten times before chilling	50
Queuing for beluga and brie	90

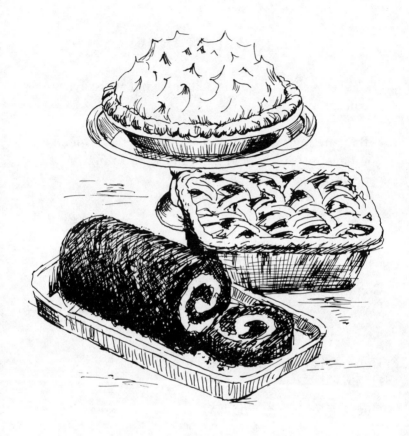

The desserts

8. JUST DESSERTS

Banana pudding • Chess pie • Pecan pie • Divinity • Peach cobbler • Sweet potato pie • Pineapple up-side-down cake

What's a meal without a mouth-watering finale? *The Beverly Hillbillies Diet* presents some of the tastiest pastries ever to cool on a window sill.

Activity	Calories burned
Shooing family out of the kitchen while goodies are cooling	125
Flinging failed pie crusts at the ceiling	175
Hulling pecans	100
Picking peaches, digging yams	345

This is real food, you say. But, you ask, can I eat all I want, anytime I want?

Of course you can. On *The Beverly Hillbillies Diet*, a no-frills weekly plan is as easy to follow as a path of crumbs to a gingerbread house.

See for yourself.

4

The Beverly Hillbillies Diet

THE BEVERLY HILLBILLIES DIET
Diet for *Week One*

	MORNING	MIDDAY	EVENING
DAY 1 *Weight*____	Grits	⟶	
DAY 2 *Weight*____	Grits	⟶	
DAY 3 *Weight*____	Grits	⟶	
DAY 4 *Weight*____	Water- melon ⟶ (If not avail- able, Grits)		
DAY 5 *Weight*____	Grits	⟶	
DAY 6 *Weight*____	Grits	⟶	
DAY 7 *Weight*____	Jack Daniel's ⟶		

After *Week One*

If you didn't know what grits were when we *started,* you sure as shootin' should *now.*

But don't go getting a knot in your rope; there's more than cereal to getting back to the basics.

(Just wanted to get your attention and help you put your plate in the proper perspective. You need to get a grip on your appetite, *not your fork.*)

Remember, you can put anything you want *on* the grits. Most of us prefer real butter and salt and pepper, but for the sake of variety you might want to take a look at butter and sugar.

CITIFIED EXERCISES

The Loud Sheet

There's no question but what this avalanche of grits and some of our menus for the weeks to come are going to be something of a shock to your city stomach.

And as sure as the good Lord made little green apples, your disposition and digestion will improve if you can get all that moaning and groaning out of your system.

So, get a big sheet of construction paper and nail it up someplace you can get at it.

Then get yourself a magic marker and write down any little ole thing that pops into your head, like,

"Damn those hateful grits!!!"

"Hells bells!!! I may be big as a barn, but who needs all this gruel!!!"

"Grits, schmits!"

THE BEVERLY HILLBILLIES DIET
Diet for *Week Two*

	MORNING	MIDDAY	EVENING
DAY 8 *Weight*___	Corn Bread & Collard Greens	$\longrightarrow$	
DAY 9 *Weight*___	Corn Bread & Mustard Greens	$\longrightarrow$	
DAY 10 *Weight*___	Corn Bread & Polk Salad	$\longrightarrow$	
DAY 11 *Weight*___	White Lightning	$\longrightarrow$	
DAY 12 *Weight*___	Corn Bread & Water-melon (if not available, Black-strap Molasses)	$\longrightarrow$	

DAY 13 *Weight*____	Moon Pies & South- ern Cham- pagne*	──────────→
DAY 14 *Weight*____	Corn Bread & Turnip Greens	──────────→

* See glossary, *s'il vous plaît*.

After *Week Two*

I can just hear you hollering now:

"Where is the Pig Group??!!"

"What the hell has happened to the Henhouse??!!"

"What went with The Pond?!?!"

Well, hold on now, big fellas and gals!

You all admit that you've been going whole hog for some little time now, so we have had to help you learn to fence in your appetite a tad.

Don't forget that the purpose of these first few weeks is too help you bust loose of city cuisine and get your body ready for Country Combining.

To do this you're going to be tying on the feedbag with Farm Foods, not Fancy Foods.

The Beverly Hillbillies Diet will work for you.

But you'll have to stick with it longer than Pat stayed in the Army.

CITIFIED EXERCISES

Affirmative Traction

Since you're basically having only greens during this phase, go ahead and weld the refrigerator door shut. You'll forget and pull on it four or five hundred times during the course of the week and will feel a whole lot better for it.

THE BEVERLY HILLBILLIES DIET
Diet for *Week Three*

	MORNING	MIDDAY	EVENING
DAY 15 *Weight*____	Pecan Pie	————————————————→	
DAY 16 *Weight*____	Peach Cobbler	————————————————→	
DAY 17 *Weight*____	Chess Pie	————————————————→	
DAY 18 *Weight*____	Divinity	————————————————→	
DAY 19 *Weight*____	Pineapple Upside- down Cake	————————————————→	
DAY 20 *Weight*____	Sweet Potato Pie	————————————————→	
DAY 21 *Weight*____	Banana Pudding	————————————————→	

After *Week Three*

Even though we hadn't said anything about it, we bet you noticed one little bitty ole thing missing from our Hillbilly menus so far: desserts.

And—tell the truth—didn't you pick up a fair portion of your more ponderous parts by satisfying that ole sweet tusk?

And you've had to do it on the sly, haven't you?

Oh yes, brothers and sisters, I can see you now. Slipping into those bakeries and cookie emporiums to fill your pockets with chocolate fantasies. Sugar-coated whatnots.

Well, nobody has to be ashamed of being partial to confections. Personally, I never met a sweetmeat I didn't like.

But hear me out: You'll never get back to the basics when you are a slave to a bonbon. And sneaking sweets can be one of the toughest city fat syndromes to break.

You must face up to your pastry dependency, and there's no time like the present.

This is the week you *Beverly Hillbillies* dieters get what you've been craving: Your just desserts.

CITIFIED EXERCISES

Rolling Over

While you've got your rolling pin down off the shelf, roll it around for ten minutes on each of the parts of yourself you especially need to reduce.

THE BEVERLY HILLBILLIES DIET
Diet for *Week Four*

	MORNING	MIDDAY	EVENING
DAY 22 *Weight*____	Black-eyed Peas	⟶	
DAY 23 *Weight*____	Fried Okra	⟶	
DAY 24 *Weight*____	Crowder Peas	⟶	
DAY 25 *Weight*____	Yellow Squash	⟶	
DAY 26 *Weight*____	Corn on the Cob	⟶	Fried Corn
DAY 27 *Weight*____	Field Peas	⟶	
DAY 28 *Weight*____	Fried Green Tomatoes	⟶	

After *Week Four*

After last week, you are probably going to jump and run at the teeniest suggestion of anything sweet to eat.

You might even feel a little queasy when some old friend calls up to say "Hi, Sugar!"

But don't fret.

This week, the Patch Food Group returns to the front of the trough. Neighbors, we've got three kinds of people-pleasin' peas, all cooked up real delicious.

And we'd like you to meet okra, those popular, furry little pods. I just know you're going to like fried okra so much you'll want to eat it at the movies instead of popcorn.

If you've never had fried tomatoes, you are in for a special taste of down-home goodness.

So get out your fatback and cornmeal and keep those hillbilly home fires burning through Week Four.

CITIFIED EXERCISES

Shuck, rattle, and roll

The time you spend in fixing meals can do double duty as you tone your torso. Put those Elvis Presley, Bill Hailey, and Jerry Lee Lewis records on the turntable and shimmy while your dinner simmers.

THE BEVERLY HILLBILLIES DIET
Diet for *Week Five*

	MORNING	MIDDAY	EVENING
DAY 29 Weight___	Huckle-berries ⟶		Frog Legs, Watercress, Baked Potato
DAY 30 Weight___	Turnip Greens ⟶		
DAY 31 Weight___	Bacon & Eggs, Sliced Tomatoes ⟶		
DAY 32 Weight___	Ham & Biscuits, Grits ⟶		
DAY 33 Weight___	Corn Bread & Buttermilk ⟶		Chicken & Dumplings
DAY 34 Weight___	Sugar Pears	Peaches	Persim-mons
DAY 35 Weight___	Apple-sauce ⟶		Applejack

After *Week Five*

This is the week you've been waiting for:

Pardner, the Pig Group, The Pond, and The Hen-house are all back in business in your dining room.

Our first month of hillbilly sensibility is beginning to pay off. Your shape is beginning to change and your kith and kin are starting to notice a change in you.

Aren't your overalls baggier than ever before?

How long has it been since you broke the settee you sat on?

You and your garden are underway. Don't let up now.

Remember, you only get to fitness by letting go of fatness.

CITIFIED EXERCISES

The Joe Bob Assignment

"Can you guess my weight?"
"Can I guess your weight?"
"I'd say she weighs about——."

Go ahead and talk to folks about your diet whenever you take a notion. Speak right up in elevators. Let them know you may live in the city but you're no slicker when it comes to noticing hips and thighs and other key city spots that might slip up and get heavy on you.

It's a fack that fitness and fatness are on everybody's mind.

Then slip your neighbor the grip and tell him ever since you started *The Beverly Hillbillies Diet* that your weight has been dropping like an anorexic at a church supper.

Suggest he run over to his neighborly bookseller and pick himself up a copy, and maybe an extra for a fat-type friend. Spread the word about the Golden Grit and reduce unsightly spread in your city friends and neighbors.

THE BEVERLY HILLBILLIES DIET
Diet for *Week Six*

	MORNING	MIDDAY	EVENING
DAY 36 *Weight*___	Black-berries	⟶	Fried Catfish, Potatoes & Onions, Hushpuppies, Sliced Tomatoes, Blackberry Cobbler
DAY 37 *Weight*___	Bacon & Eggs	⟶	Fried Chicken, Green Beans, Mashed Potatoes, Gravy, Biscuits, Chocolate Icebox Pie
DAY 38 *Weight*___	Bananas	⟶	Cold Chicken, Bread & Butter Pickles, Three Bean Salad, Ambrosia
DAY 39 *Weight*___	Dew-berries	⟶	Porkchops, Crowder Peas, Green Tomato Pickles, Turnip Greens, Corn Sticks

DAY 40 *Weight*___	Figs ⟶	Barbecued Spareribs, Bread & Butter, Cole Slaw, Baked Beans, Coconut Cake
DAY 41 *Weight*___	Brains & Eggs ⟶	Baked Ham, Deviled Eggs, Potato Salad, Homemade Ice Cream
DAY 42 *Weight*___	Flapjacks ⟶	Baked Hen, Dressing, Green Beans, Candied Yams, Black-Bottom Pie

After *Week Six*

You are home free now.

Each and every one of *The Fabulous Beverly Hillbillies Diet Food Groups* is making a beeline to your place at the table.

You are proving that by using common sense alongside silverware you can get back to a sensible size and stay there.

Now, when the plates are being passed 'round this week, remember: You don't have to get all that's coming to you at just that one sitting.

There's no call to overdo it today because you might just run across a blueberry muffin down the road a bit.

Don't inhale every morsel the minute it is set in front of you. Today's fried chicken dinner is tomorrow's cold supper. Barbecued spareribs and black-eyed peas are even better the second time around. Same with dressing and gravy.

So take your time.

Butter that second biscuit slow and easy.

You're on your way to Country Combining.

CITIFIED EXERCISES

Food Sassing

Think back to the days when you couldn't get through the barn door. What were you eating so much of that got you into trouble in the first place? Get another sheet of construction paper and draw pictures of those foods and tell them off. Go ahead. Sass that food:

"Napoleon, I lied; I never really loved you."

"White truffles, you are nothing but white trash!!"

"Hey, lasagna! Your sister sleeps with truck drivers!!"

5

Country
Combining
Explained

COUNTRY COMBINING EXPLAINED

Now you have overcome the dread pasta dependency and mastered our *Hillbilly Basic Food Groups.*

Your hips have returned to the straight and narrow instead of the high and wide.

Your waistline is under control—and under a normal belt instead of a length of garden hose—so you can now go barreling down the healthy highway of Country Combining.

At this point you can combine simple country foods with some of your leftover citified culinary idiosyncrasies. Feel free to combine some of the basics with your old palate persuasions.

For example:

HILLBILLY	ITALIAN	JEWISH	FRENCH	ENGLISH
Grits	Gritticotti	Tsimis Grits	Grits Bechamel	Shepherd's Grits
Collard Greens	Zuppa di Collardi	Collard Kreplach	Collard Veronique	Collard Pie
Catfish	Catfish tonnata	Catfish-knish	Catfish a la Creeque	Catfish Albert
Corn Bread	Corn-meal Misto	Corn-Bread Kishka	Crois-sants de Corn	Corn-scones
BBQ Ribs	Pigglia e Fiena	———	Pig au Feu	Pig Well-ington

Still, don't forget to heft things other than your fork.

SOME HILLBILLY TIPS TO HELP YOU LOSE WEIGHT

1. **Sit 'way back from the table.**
   The harder it is to reach your food, the less likely you are to overeat.

2. **Slow down.**
   Take it easy. You're chewing so fast your mouth is nothing but a blur. Don't jump on your food like a duck on a June bug.

3. **Take smaller helpings.**
   Don't put anything on your plate that is bigger than a pocketwatch.

4. **Forget about seconds.**

5. **Tie fishing weights to your fork.**
   That should slow you up a bit. Or you might try using one of those fancy Swiss army knives and just pulling out the fork when it's time to take a bite and then put it back and then pull it out when you need it again and so forth.

6. **Wear overalls.**
   If you are not all slicked up, people will be less likely to invite you out to those fancy places for lunch or dinner. Overalls will camouflage your bulk and remind you to concentrate on losing weight. Finally, you'll have a big assortment of pockets to fill with Emergency Grits Packets.*

7. **Subways.**
   Take the express and walk back to your local stop.

---

* See recipe (that's right, you can turn some pages; interrupting yourself burns up lots of calories).

8. **Tape an oatmeal box around your elbow.**
A cousin of mine in Nashville who used to cause eclipses used this trick. It made eating a whole lot more challenging, and she lost a lot of weight.

9. **Eliminate phrases.**
"Pass the ——," "à la mode," "Whopper,"and "don't mind if I do" must be stricken from your vocabulary.

10. **Go to the well.**
Drink at least one glass of water for every five bites you take. That way, what with fastening and unfastening your overalls and running to the john, you just won't have all that much time left to feed your face.

11. **Stretch your legs.**
So many city people just settle unto haunch heaven. They can't do anything *but* sit behind desks, in front of typewriters or bridge tables. Is it any wonder the body bottoms out?
Take a walk after dinner. Make it a daily constitutional.
If you live in a real city, like New York, you may even have a reason to run a little ways.
If you live in Beverly Hills, this will mean exchanging your limo for shoes, but it will be novel.
And remember, you'll be wearing your overalls so no one will recognize you.

12. **Use plastic forks and knives.**
Bear down.

13. **Escalators.**
Just because you are already moving is no excuse not to walk.

14. **Move your wastepaper basket 'way away from your desk.**

    You'll probably miss it most of the time and will have to get up, go over, and pick up all those wads. Marvelous for the waistline.

15. **Pick up your date in a wheelbarrow.**

    She will admire your strength and resourcefulness. Most couples agree it's more fun than a rickshaw. The wheelbarrow is also the perfect vehicle when you hit the sales at Neiman's or I. Magnin.

16. **Start a job jar.**

    When you've finished all your chores, you won't be chubby.

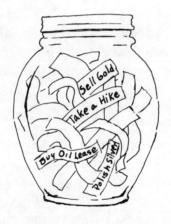

6
As the World Churns

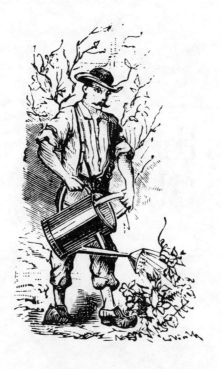

Weeding the garden

BEVERLY HILLBILLIES DIET EXERCISES FOR SPECIFIC AREAS

In addition to cutting back on your intake, you are going to need to increase your output. Or, as we say down home, shake a leg. Look alive. Get a move on.

Depending on which part of your body needs a tad of trimming, we have some ideas on how to whittle those thighs and other things down to size.

FOR THE WAIST

HILLBILLY ACTIVITIES	CITY SUBSTITUTIONS (as necessary)
Cotton picking	Litter picking
Weeding the garden	Weeding the median
Splitting kindling	Cleaning out the attic
Pick stones up out of the pasture	Pick up movie stubs for tax returns
Sickeling weeds	Practicing iron shots for an hour
Waving at the Charles Chips man	Washing all your windows

FOR THE UPPER ARMS

HILLBILLY ACTIVITIES	CITY SUBSTITUTIONS (as necessary)
Churning	Pull ups on transit straps
Putting in fence posts	Polish silver service
Hanging out wash	Rehanging every picture in the house
Forking over compost pile	Forking over margin call
Rolling biscuits	Rowing to Catalina

FOR THE CHIN & FACIAL MUSCLES

HILLBILLY ACTIVITIES	CITY SUBSTITUTIONS (as necessary)
Hog calling	Buying an oil lease
Talking over the back fence	Negotiating distribution deal with Coppola
Intense quilting bee	Meeting with co-op board

FOR THE BOTTOM AND LEGS

HILLBILLY ACTIVITIES	CITY SUBSTITUTIONS (as necessary)
Buckdancing	An evening at 54
Lively ramble around the north forty	Lively ramble around Benedict Canyon
Clod kicking	Pigeon kicking

CAST-IRON CALISTHENICS

The Beverly Hillbillies Diet eliminates the need to buy expensive and space-consuming exercise machinery.

Simply by using three major kitchen appliances, you will be able to increase dramatically the effectiveness of these traditional citified exercises.

The Skillet   *The Griddle*   *The Corn-Sticks Pan*

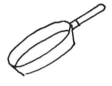 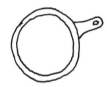 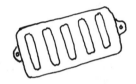

SIT-UPS: Strap corn-stick pan to forehead.
Proceed with sit-ups as usual.

LEG LIFTS: Tie griddle to ankle for improved toning.

PUSH-UPS: Stack skillet, griddle, and corn-sticks pan on back.
Proceed with push-ups as usual.

CHIN-UPS: Put corn-sticks pan, griddle, and skillet down your sweatpants. Your chin-ups will work harder than ever.

PUMPING CAST IRON

1. Attach cast-iron utensils to broom stick or mop handle.
2. Lie down on ironing board.
3. And one, and two, and one, and two . . .

ALL 'ROUND CONDITIONING EXERCISES

Pig Flipping.
This is an excellent torso firmer and reducer. First thing is to catch the varmint. Then grip firmly under the forelegs and give him a nice back flip. Catch the pig and repeat. A basset hound may be substituted.

Melon Hefting.
As an out-of-shape beginner, you'll probably start at the honeydew level. Get two big ones. Place a honeydew in each hand; lift and lower them several hundred times. Your goal is to work up to watermelons. Keep your eyes open for other hefting opportunities, such as hams at Easter, trees at Christmas, or babies any old time.

Bale Vaulting.
Cotton bales are best because they are so big, but bales of hay are fine, too. Haul a couple of dozen over to your yard, set yourself up a course, and have at it. Piano benches can be substituted for bales and you could even work up to foreign cars. Fire hydrants are acceptable as are large dogs, but you must be quick.

Cat Putting.
This is a variation of the shot put on account of cats are usually handier. Again, don't overlook those seasonal putting opportunities, among which we recommend the turkey put, the pumpkin put, and the very invigorating bunny put.

Tree Climbing.
We have all done this as children; it is an ageless activity which provides fine conditioning for adults as well. Take it easy at first (do not start with one of the palms on Sunset). Practice alone. You will dramatically improve muscle tone and will also win bets from flabby friends.

CORRECTIVE MEASURES

Let's face it: Much of life consists of fixing things that have gone wrong.

So it goes with vittles.

The Beverly Hillbillies Diet prepares you for these "I overdid it" occasions with some home remedies to dining-out indiscretions.

Here are several ways to make amends for getting carried away at the buffet.

The Okra Offensive.
Stew a bushel of okra. Serve until it's gone and all the pounds you picked up on your prosciutto fiasco will be gone with it.

The Carrot Cure-all.
Measure your waist. The number of inches you are around is the number of orange roots you'll be crunching the day after your bagel binge.

The Tomato Vendetta.
Mason Williams originated this country concept of eating ten tomatoes each meal for two days after straying from the paths of dietiousness.

SOUTHERN INSPIRATIONAL READING FOR BEVERLY HILLBILLIES DIETERS

When you just start out on a diet, it doesn't hurt to know that even famous people have had to pass through the Dark Night of the Fork.

It is a little-known fact that a number of well-known southern authors suffered from weight problems after they got away from the Chitlin Belt.

Some had such fat fingers they could hardly hit one typewriter key at a time. They have asked to remain anonymous but you will recognize these descriptions of their fat-phase works-in-progress.

Delta Wedding Cake. A southern family searching for a long-lost recipe for angel food cake is rescued by a visiting cousin who not only reconstructs the recipe but brings with her forty egg whites and a funnel pan with a removable rim.

Free Deliverance (with minimum order of $10). A provocative tale of four bachelors' survival struggle in the rough and tumble world of late night carry-out restaurants.

All The Chef's Men. The inspiring saga of a Louisiana short-order cook. Mastering the kitchen politics of the finest restaurants in the South, he at last reaches Galatoire's. As his fame grows, he sets his apron for San Souci in Washington but is assassinated by a group of vengeful bus boys.

A Good Flan Is Hard to Find. A family traveling through the south in search of household help. Alas, no candidate's references satisfy the grandmother of the family. The matriarch eventually jumps off a bridge when the family hires a Cuban housekeeper.

All the Way Home for Dessert. The father drinks but is at last rescued from the curse of alcoholism when his gifts at making puff pastry are discovered.

Light Lunch in August. A rambling stream of calorie consciousness. A Mississippi family's dramatic history as told through their menus for several years. Readers will forever debate the haunting question, did the hostess make the mousse herself?

Night of the Barbecued Iguana. A minister who's been giving away wine all his life finally starts to hit the sauce himself. But, his beaujolais-based barbecue sauce makes the island parish's picnics the best ever.

Perhaps you will also be driven to inspiration, just like these fine former fatties.

SIDE EFFECTS OF THE BEVERLY HILLBILLIES DIET

- Marion D. formed a quilting bee to reduce fat fore-arms and fingers. Her group now sells the quilts, using the proceeds to stock a trout farm.

- Dr. Michael W. saved countless waistlines by developing a hollandaise vaccination.

- Henry L. made a fortune selling cornmeal futures.

- Forrest W., a department store magnate, increased sales 22 percent by installing Overalls Boutiques in all his stores.

- Ellen C. married Walter K. after watching him browbeat Balducci's into carrying crowder peas.

- Rob B. was given a lifetime gift certificate at Gucci's after suggesting they sell alligator brogans.

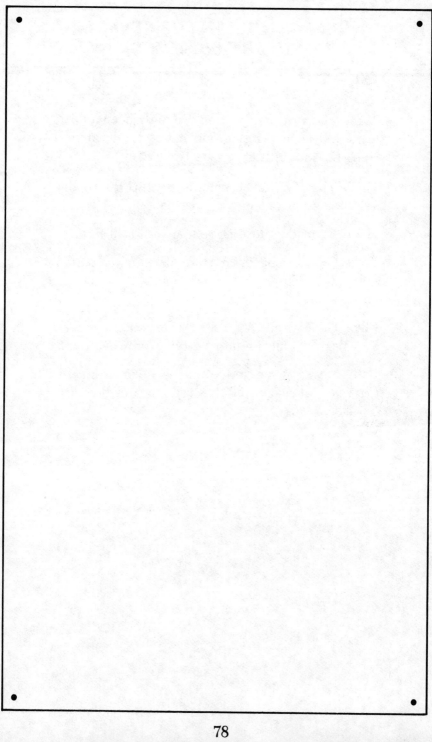

7

Questions and Answers

Q: I can't stop accepting luncheon invitations. What should I do?
A: Make arrangements to walk back and forth when you are invited to lunch. A nice hike from Bel Air to the Orangery or from Bronxville to Le Cirque will do you a world of good. You'll see that a bowl of leftover greens with some cold corn bread can be mighty good eating.

Q: Doesn't your diet assume a lot of acreage to follow the regimen?
A: This is a big country. There's bound to be a park or a field or a zoo or a quiet street near you even if you don't have a good-sized spread of your own. You don't have to live on the Ponderosa to stay on *The Beverly Hillbillies Diet*. If you don't have a park or an arboretum in your town, maybe you ought to endow one.

(Ingenuity uses 300 calories an hour. Be clever for two hours about how to buckle down and then you *can* have a peach fried pie!)

Q: When I eat alone, I just shovel it in because there's no one to talk to. Any suggestions?
A: You are probably old enough now to read at the table. There is some danger of dropping your book in the salad dressing but that's better than giving in to lonely fat. When eating alone you need to have something on your mind other than your plate and your palate.

Q: I have heard that the kiwi contains an enzyme essential to the utilization of the weight-loss vitamins M and N. Is this true?
A: The kiwi is a little bird that makes shoe polish, not anything you need to eat a lot of. Besides, kiwis are kind of cute and there are not many of them left.

Q: What should I do when I'm invited to my boss's house for dinner and everything is fattening?

A: When you know you're going to be tying on the feedbag at suppertime, you can't take on the entire Pig Group at lunch. It's not the day for flapjacks and sorghum at sun-up, either. If you want to enjoy yourself at dinner—and in this case, keep your job—you can't go whole hog all day.

Q: Is it true that alcohol is fattening? After a few belts I don't feel so fat anymore.

A: You may have an idea there. Have a few more and you'll probably even sleep through dinner.

Q: When I'm happy, I eat. Is there any hope for me?

A: Could be a little misery is what you need. Stick to those pithy store-bought tomatoes for a week.

Q: I've been trying to stay on my diet for a long time, but I get no support from my family. They just say, "Mom, there's more of you to love."

A: Sounds to me like they aim to keep you kitchen bound. Shake a leg, honey and get away from that stove.

Q: I have put on weight because I eat street food on my way to the train station after work. How can I kick the Sabrett's habit?

A: Fix up some Emergency Grit packets to carry in your overalls at all times.

8
Miss Ruby's Recipes

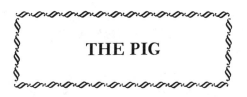

THE PIG

BARBECUED SPARERIBS

Figure about a pound or maybe a little more per person, because these are favorites of everybody's.

First thing is to plunge the ribs—which you ought to cut crossways so they are of a manageable size—into boiling water for three or four minutes. This cooks them part-way and also gets rid of any unnecessary fat.

Then take them outdoors over the grill or the pit on a spit and cook them for about an hour over slow heat.

Baste every ten minutes with our Barbecue Sauce.

Cook another ten minutes and baste every time you get a chance.

THE BEVERLY HILLBILLIES DIET
BARBECUE SAUCE

1½ cups vegetable oil
½ quart vinegar
2 cans tomato sauce
2 bottles catsup
½ pound butter
½ bottle Tabasco
1 box celery seed

½ tablespoon salt
3   cloves garlic, finely chopped
3 large onions, chopped or grated
¼ teaspoon black pepper
12 lemons
Worcestershire sauce

Combine all these good things (except lemons and Worcestershire sauce) and mix real well. Put on the stove and bring to a boil.

Remove from heat and add half the bottle of Worcestershire sauce and the juice of the lemons.

This sauce will keep well in your icebox for some time or you can freeze it. It is especially good with chicken, porkchops, or barbecued ribs.

PORKCHOPS FOR THE PREACHER
(or whatever company's coming for dinner)

4 porkchops
Flour
1 clove garlic, minced
Salt
Pepper
4 Irish potatoes, peeled
   and sliced

2 large onions, sliced
1½ cups sour cream
½ teaspoon dry mustard
1½ teaspoons salt
Cooking oil

Preheat your oven to 350°F.

Trim any excess fat from your chops and roll them in flour.

Brown the chops and the garlic in hot oil over medium heat.

Season with salt and pepper.

Put the sliced potatoes in a casserole and cover them with the chops. Separate the onion slices into rings and put them on top of the chops.

Blend the sour cream, the salt, and the mustard. Pour this mixture over the chops, potatoes, and onions.

Bake an hour and a half. This gives you a little time to check the job jar, if you've got everything else ready for dinner.

This will serve four of you.

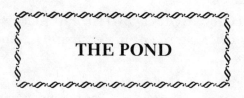

THE POND

FRIED CATFISH

Catch, clean, and skin a catfish. Toss in a paper bag with some cornmeal seasoned with salt and pepper. Fry in a skillet of hot fat until golden brown.

Save the drippings for hushpuppies (see page 100).

Depending on your appetite after a full day at the pond, plan on about half a pound of catfish for each serving.

This meal is a good opportunity to do arm exercises while you talk about the One That Got Away.

BAKED BASS WITH CORN BREAD STUFFING

4½–5 pound bass
Salt and pepper
Bacon, 4 strips, fried
½ stick sweet butter

One lemon
Worcestershire sauce
Extra bass head

Clean the fish well; make sure you get all the scales off. Boil the extra head or small filet to make stock.

Lay an oiled cheesecloth in your baking pan.

Gash the fish about every two inches or so. Salt and pepper well and then place small pieces of bacon in the gashes.

Baste while cooking with the stock which you have mixed with the juice of one lemon, the butter, Worcestershire, salt, and pepper to your taste.

Bake in a preheated 450°F oven for ten minutes per pound.

Corn Bread Stuffing

1½ cup sliced celery, sautéed in butter
1 large onion sautéed in butter
2 cups water
3 cups corn bread crumbs
Salt and pepper to taste

After you have sautéed the onion and celery, add the water and boil until tender. Pour this over the corn bread crumbs and season to taste with salt and pepper.

Fill the fish with stuffing and if you have any left over put it in the pan around the fish and it will help keep him moist while he cooks.

This baking time means you have a chance to catch up on your side-straddle hops.

The fish will serve four good eaters generously.

FROG LEGS

Catch and clean as many frogs as you need. Separate the legs from the bodies. Rinse again, then wipe the frog legs dry. Then get three bowls ready as follows:

Bowl A. A shallow bowl filled with flour seasoned with salt and pepper.

Bowl B. A mixture of slightly beaten egg diluted with a little dab of milk for each egg you use. Stir the milk and egg together about a dozen times but not so much that it gets foamy.

Bowl C. Sift some bread crumbs and season with salt and pepper. Figure not quite a heaping handful for every egg you use.

First, flour each leg in Bowl A. Pat it lightly from one hand to the other to shake loose any excess flour.

Next, slip the floured frog leg into the egg-milk mixture in Bowl B so it's all nice and coated. Let any excess drip back off.

Finally, place the leg in the crumbs in Bowl C. Be sure they stick all over.

Put the legs on your dish drainer and let them dry for about half an hour or so while you run in place on the porch. Then fry in hot fat until golden brown.

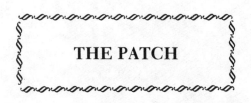

THE PATCH

GREENS
(Turnip, Collard, or Mustard Greens)

Cook a fair-sized piece of fat back or salt pork in boiling water for an hour or so.

Meanwhile, wash the greens *several times* to remove all soil.

Add to the salt pork and cook until tender.

You'll have time to work in 40 or 50 sit-ups.

Then you *can* add turnips, sliced up, about fifteen minutes before the greens have finished cooking.

FRIED OKRA

Wash the little okra pods well. Slice off the stem ends and toss. Slice the rest of the pod into pieces no bigger than a quarter of an inch. Toss the slices in cornmeal to which you have added salt and pepper.

Heat up just a little bit of oil in your skillet and add the okra. Fry for about ten minutes or until crispy.

Drain on a paper towel or the real estate section or the paper and then transfer to your serving dish.

FRIED CORN

Heat in your cast-iron skillet: A little dab of water, some salt and pepper, and a chunk of butter. Cut the kernels of fresh, tender corn into the skillet and cook slowly for about fifteen minutes.

THE HENHOUSE AND OLD BOSSY

SOUTHERN PSEUDO SOUFFLÉ

1 stick sweet butter, at room temperature
10 slices white enriched bread, with crusts removed
3 eggs
2 cups milk
½ pound mild Cheddar cheese, grated

Grease a round two quart casserole with butter. Put on sweatpants. Butter the slices of bread and cut into little, bitty squares. Put a layer of bread cubes into the bottom of the casserole, then cover with a layer of cheese. Repeat layering like this until all ingredients are used up. Then blend the eggs and milk and pour over the whole thing. Let all this sit in the refrigerator overnight. Bake at 275°F (preheated) 45 minutes while you jog down to the garden and pick some corn for dinner.

This will serve six to eight of you.

CHICKEN AND DUMPLINGS

1 large hen   Salt
2 tablespoon butter   pepper

Cut up the hen and cover with water in a kettle. Add butter, salt, and pepper to taste. Simmer until tender. Remove the hen.

Bring the liquid to a boil and add your dumplings.

Dumplings

2 cups plain flour   1 teaspoon salt
¾ cup warm water

Combine the flour salt and water. Roll the dough on floured waxed paper as thin as you can, a little bit at a time. Cut the dough into strips about an inch wide and about four inches long. Add a few at a time to the boiling hen stock. Continue until all dumplings have been dropped into kettle.

While the dumplings are cooking, tear the hen into pieces and remove most of the larger bones. After all the dumplings have been cooked, return the hen to the stock. Cover and cook over low heat for fifteen minutes.

This is a good time to do some leg lifts.

Serve at once. This should feed about six folks.

SOUTHERN FRIED CHICKEN

1 fryer (3–3½ pound)   Salt
1 egg   Pepper
1 cup flour   Shortening or vegetable
⅓ cup of milk   oil

Wash the chicken and cut it into pieces.
Combine the egg and milk in a flatish bowl.
Salt, pepper, then flour each piece of chicken.
Dip into the egg mixture and back into the flour.
Pour the oil or melt the shortening into the skillet to a depth of about two inches. Heat to medium-high and add chicken pieces. Cook covered, turning twice as each piece browns. When all pieces are browned completely, replace cover, and reduce to low heat for fifteen minutes.
Drain on a brown paper grocery bag.
This should serve four or five people.

SCRAMBLED EGGS

Break the eggs and add a little salt and pepper. Most people can handle at least an egg and a half per serving.

Then add a little heavy cream.

Then *strain* the mixture into a heated, buttered skillet. Cook slowly. Stir only two or three times with a whisk.

Don't forget that the eggs continue cooking on the way to the table.

After you've cleaned up the dishes, do fifteen minutes of cast-iron calisthenics (see our section on Pumping Cast Iron, page 71).

FRESH GAME ALTERNATIVES TO THE HENHOUSE GROUP

What could be more southern than shooting for the table? If the season is open and you have some luck, these are delicious.

COUNTRY QUAIL

Clean your birds and wash them well *(game birds should never be skinned)*. Dry them off. Roll the quail in flour with salt and pepper.

In a cast-iron skillet, bring vegetable oil to medium high heat. Submerge each bird completely. Keep the oil at an even temperature. Cook for ten minutes or until golden brown, taking care not to break the skin.

Figure on a bird or two per person.

COUNTRY SQUIRREL OR RABBIT

Clean and wash well. Cut into pieces like you would a chicken. Put in a cast-iron skillet and add enough water to cover.

Put the lid on the skillet and cook over medium heat for thirty minutes. Take the lid off and add salt and pepper and a little bit of oil. Cook down until brown.

After you've taken up the game you can make a delicious cream gravy right there in the same pan to go with your rice and potatoes and biscuits.

Just add 1½ tablespoons of flour, a cup of milk, a half cup of water, and a dab more salt and pepper to the drippings. Stir all around over medium heat until the gravy happens.

A full day of hunting to get a full game bag is exercise enough in itself. Enjoy your supper; almost everybody can eat two or three pieces.

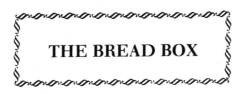

THE BREAD BOX

CORN BREAD

2 tablespoons cooking oil
2 cups white self-rising cornmeal
1⅓ cups milk (buttermilk is best)
1 egg, slightly beaten

Preheat oven to 450°F.

Oil your cast-iron skillet, cornstick or muffin pan and put in the oven until hot. Combine your milk and egg. Add to meal. Stir until smooth. Pour batter into pan.

Bake 20 to 25 minutes for a pan of corn bread.

Bake 15 to 20 minutes for sticks or muffins. Makes a dozen.

While the bread is baking, do 25 side-straddle hops.

Note. As you go through life, you may meet folks who will suggest to you that corn bread can be made either with yellow cornmeal or with a little bit of sugar in the batter. Stay away from these people; they are agents of the devil.

HUSHPUPPIES

Make corn bread batter. Add some minced onion and minced bell pepper. Make into golf-ball-sized wads. Use the fat you just used to cook your fish and fry the hush puppies until golden brown.

CHEESE GRITS

1 cup grits
1½ cups sharp Cheddar cheese, grated
½ cup sweet butter
½ cup milk (evaporated is best)
2 eggs, well beaten
Tabasco to taste

Preheat oven to 350°F.

Cook the grits according to package directions. Stir in cheese, butter, milk, eggs, and dash of Tabasco. Keep on cooking over low heat until all the cheese is melted while doing leg lifts off to one side. Pour mixture into a 2-quart greased casserole or baking dish. Bake about an hour. Serves six.

EMERGENCY GRITS PACKETS

Fix yourself a batch of grits. Let them cool down just a bit and then ladle out a half cup or so into plastic food bags.

Add a little butter and salt and pepper. Then tie the baggie closed with some good, stout kitchen twine.

Keep these in the pockets of your overalls when the urge to munch overtakes you.

SPOON BREAD

Step One

1½ teaspoon sugar
1½ teaspoon salt
1 cup cornmeal
4 tablespoons sweet butter

Mix sugar, salt, and meal. Melt butter in 1⅓ cups boiling water. Pour water over mixture and mix in well. Let cool overnight (or for four hours) at room temperature. Just before going to bed, do 40 deep knee-bends.

Step Two

3 eggs
1 tablespoon baking powder
1½ cups hot milk
(or cream if you want a richer texture)

Preheat oven to 350°F.

Grease a 2-quart casserole with butter. Beat eggs and baking powder and add to previous mixture. Pour into casserole and bake for 35 to 45 minutes. Serves four with second helpings.

BANANA BREAD

¼ cup shortening
2 cups flour
3 ripe bananas
1 teaspoon sour milk
1 teaspoon baking soda, sifted into flour
¼ teaspoon salt, sifted into flour
1 cup sugar
2 eggs
½ cup pecans or walnuts

Preheat oven to 350°F.

Cream sugar and shortening. Add beaten eggs. Crush bananas well with a fork, then add to mixture. Then add sour milk. Mix. Then add the flour. Mix well.

Bake for 35 to 45 minutes.

Lie down on the kitchen floor and practice scissor kicks while you're waiting.

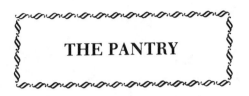

THE PANTRY

GREEN TOMATO & SWEET PEPPER PICKLES

Firm green tomatoes	Canning salt
Firm bell peppers	Water
Firm hot peppers	1½ cups vinegar

Wash the tomatoes. Cut off the ends and slice or quarter.

Do the same thing with the bell peppers. Pack an assortment of the three peppers—using hot peppers according to your taste and tolerance—to within an inch of the top of each *sterilized jar.*

Put a teaspoon of canning salt on the top of each jar.

Then mix a cup of water with the vinegar and bring them just to a boil. Pour this water and vinegar mixture over the peppers and seal well, according to the manufacturer's directions. Some people add a clove of garlic.

Store one jar at a time on a high shelf you have to stretch to reach.

PEAR PRESERVES

Peel, quarter, and core enough pears to cover the bottom of a large, heavy pan. Generously dust with sugar. Alternate layers of pears and sugar until the pan is filled. Cover pan. Let it sit out on the kitchen table overnight.

Next morning, put the pan on the stove and bring the mixture to a hard boil while you are stirring it well.

Reduce the heat and cook slowly until the syrup is like honey. Add some lemon slices when the syrup has thickened.

Pour into *sterilized jars* and seal lids tightly, according to manufacturer's directions.

Store in a cool, dark place you have to stretch or bend over to reach.

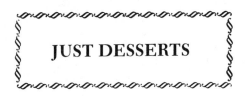

JUST DESSERTS

PECAN PIE

3 eggs
1 cup dark brown sugar
1 cup Karo light corn
 syrup
1 teaspoon vanilla

1 tablespoon sweet butter,
 melted
1 cup chopped pecans
1 9-inch baked pastry crust
 (crust should be light
 brown)

Beat eggs until light. Add sugar gradually. Add remaining ingredients and blend well. Pour into pastry shell. Bake about one hour in a preheated 350°F oven.

Get ready for this delicious dessert by doing 30 situps.

This will make your traditional nine-inch-type pie. You can figure on about eight slices.

CHESS PIE

6 egg yolks, well beaten
1 cup sugar
¾ cup sweet butter, at room temperature
1 teaspoon vanilla
1 teaspoon cornmeal
3 tablespoons cream

Preheat oven to 450°F.

Beat ingredients until well blended. Pour into un-baked pie crust. Reduce oven temperature to 350°F. Bake until golden brown and custard is well set, about 30 minutes.

You can check it every five or ten minutes while you are running laps around the house.

This will bake up into a nine-inch pie, which provides you and your happy group with about eight slices.

BANANA PUDDING

5 or 6 medium-sized bananas, sliced
Juice of one lemon
2 tablespoons sugar
3 tablespoons flour
1 whole egg plus 3 egg yolks
2 cups milk
½ teaspoon vanilla extract
Vanilla wafers, one box

Soak sliced bananas in lemon juice for about 15 minutes. Then set aside.

Combine the sugar and flour in the top of a double boiler.

Mix in eggs and milk.

Cook over boiling water, stirring constantly until thickened. Remove from heat. Stir in vanilla.

In a deep casserole dish, make layers of custard, vanilla wafers, and sliced bananas, in that order. The top and bottom layers should be custard.

Bake in a preheated 425°F oven for 5 to 10 minutes. Do 10 chin-ups.

Serve hot or cold.

Makes six to eight satisfying servings.

Note: As you see there are three loose egg whites left over from this recipe, and if you feel strongly about it, go ahead and do meringue for the top.

Get your egg whites to room temperature. Beat the

three of them wildly until they are foamy. Put in a tea-spoon of vanilla extract. Keep on beating while you add, a teaspoon at a time, ¾ cup of sifted powdered sugar. When the mixture is standing in stiff peaks, it is ready to be plopped on the pudding and baked at 325°F for about ten minutes, or until peaks are golden.

PEACH COBBLER

1 batch of biscuit dough (package directions or heirloom
 recipe)
4 to 6 ripe peaches, peeled and sliced
1 egg
2 tablespoons flour
⅔ cup sugar
⅓ cup sweet butter, melted
Cinnamon

Make enough biscuit dough to cover the top of a
deep-dish–ovenproof bowl; put aside.

Fill the bowl with peach slices. Combine the egg with
the flour, sugar, and butter. Blend real well and pour
over the peaches. Sprinkle with cinnamon.

Cover with biscuit dough and bake in a preheated
425°F for about half an hour or until the dough is a
crispy, golden brown. Cool awhile and serve; this is even
more delicious with some nice vanilla ice cream.

This cobbler will provide six to eight servings.

SWEET POTATO PIE

1 nine-inch pie crust, unbaked
2 cups sweet potatoes (white), mashed
1 cup milk
1½ cups sugar
2 eggs, well beaten
¼ cup melted butter
1 teaspoon vanilla extract
½ teaspoon lemon extract
1 teaspoon nutmeg
½ teaspoon salt

Blend filling ingredients in a mixer or food processor at medium speed. Pour into the crust and bake about an hour at 300°F until the middle of the pie is firm. Cool. Serves six to eight happy guests.

DIVINITY

1 cup boiling water
¾ cup Karo light corn syrup
3 cups sugar
Pinch of salt
2 egg whites, well beaten
1 cup pecans, chopped
1 teaspoon vanilla

Heat water, syrup, sugar, and salt to soft-ball stage (234°F on a candy thermometer). Add half of the mixture, a tablespoon at a time, to egg whites, heating constantly. Continue cooking remaining syrup until it reaches the crack stage (270°F) and pour into egg mixture and continue beating until high gloss changes to dull look. Fold in pecans and vanilla and drop by the spoonful on wax paper. Have boiling water ready in case candy sets too fast. Add 2 or 3 drops to make it creamy, if necessary, as it is spooned onto wax paper. Cool and cut. Makes 48 pieces.

Note: Don't try to make this delicacy on a humid day; try as you might, you just won't be able to make it set.

PECAN SOUFFLÉ

¼ cup sweet butter
¼ cup flour
½ teaspoon salt
1 cup milk
3 eggs, separated
½ cup sugar

1 cup pecans, finely
chopped
1 teaspoon vanilla
1 cup cream, whipped
½ teaspoon grated lemon
rind

Melt your butter in a double boiler. Stir in the flour and salt. Gradually add milk, stirring constantly until you have got a thick paste.

Combine the beaten egg yolks, sugar, pecans, and vanilla, mixing well.

To this add the butter mixture and stir until it is well blended.

Beat the egg whites until they are stiff as a board and fold in. This is wonderful for toning arms and shoulders.

Turn all of this into a buttered soufflé dish or casserole.

Place in a pan of hot water and bake at 350°F for 45 to 60 minutes or until the thing is set.

Serve right away with the whipped cream to which you have added the lemon rind.

This little honey serves six of you.

PINEAPPLE UPSIDE-DOWN CAKE

½ cup sweet butter plus 1 tablespoon
1 cup brown sugar, packed
1 cup pecans, chopped
1 8-ounce can of pineapple slices, drained
1 cup cake flour
1 teaspoon double-acting baking powder
4 egg yolks
1 teaspoon vanilla
1 cup sugar
4 egg whites

Melt ½ cup butter in a cast-iron skillet. Add the brown sugar and cook over low heat until melted, stirring each and every minute. Take the pan off the stove and add the pecans. Then arrange those pretty yellow rings on the bottom of the skillet in the sugar and pecan mixture.

Now make the cake batter by sifting the cake flour. Then, sift it again with the baking powder. In another bowl beat the egg yolks; then add the extra tablespoon of butter and the vanilla. In yet another bowl sift the sugar. And, in your last bowl, take those egg whites and whip them until they are stiff but not dry. Fold in the sifted sugar, a tablespoon at a time; then add the yolk mixture, and, finally, the sifted flour, a spoonful or two at a time.

Bake the cake in a preheated 325°F oven for half an

hour. Check for doneness—does the cake spring back when you touch it?

Turn the cake out of the pan, cool, and don't turn it over; the whole idea is to serve it upside-down, right?

This recipe will give you eight pretty servings.

COCONUT CAKE

¾ sweet butter
1½ cups sugar
1 teaspoon vanilla extract
3¾ cups sifted cake flour
4 teaspoons baking powder
½ teaspoon salt
1 cup milk
4 egg whites
2 cups grated coconut
1 recipe White Mountain icing

Sift together the flour, baking powder and salt. In another bowl, cream the butter gradually adding 1 cup sugar, beating until the mixture is very smooth. Stir in the extracts. Add the flour mixture alternately with the milk, beginning and ending with flour.

Beat the egg whites with half a cup of sugar until firm; fold into the batter—be gentle but thorough.

Divide the batter into three 8-inch cake pans which have been buttered and lightly floured. Bake the three layers in a 350°F oven for about 25 minutes, or until they test done by springing back when touched by your finger. Cool the layers on your dish rack for about five minutes; remove them from the pans and let them cool completely.

Spread the layers with White Mountain icing and grated coconut and assemble the cake. Then, ice the sides and top. Sprinkle the top with more grated coconut, and go ahead and pat a generous coating around the sides.

This old-fashioned goody will make any dinner party an instant hit. (It serves about eight.)

WHITE MOUNTAIN ICING

3 cups sugar
1 cup water
¼ teaspoon cream of tartar
3 egg whites
Pinch of salt
½ teaspoon vanilla extract
½ teaspoon almond extract

Get out your best saucepan. Cook together the sugar, water, and cream of tartar until the syrup spins a long thread when dropped from a spoon.

Beat the egg whites with salt until stiff; pour the syrup in a very thin slow stream into the egg whites, beating briskly until the icing holds a definite shape.

Flavor the icing with the extracts and use to fill and ice coconut cake.

PRALINES

3 cups light brown sugar, firmly packed
¼ cup water
1 tablespoon sweet butter
1 cup pecans

Cook the sugar, water, and butter in a saucepan until a bit dropped in cold water forms a soft ball. Quickly stir in the pecans and take the pan off the heat. Keep on stirring until the mixture becomes so thick and dark that you can't see through it.

Drop the mix from a spoon onto wax paper, forming small patties.

This will make you about two dozen pralines and a lot of friends.

9
Glossary and Keepsake Collection

GLOSSARY

Brogans. The important shoe, semi-high-top-type, for the well-heeled hillbilly about town. In patent for evening wear.

Country mile. How far you ought to walk each and every day.

Fack. The absolute truth.

Feedbag. What you've been tying on too often.

Hongry. What you get when you have put off eating.

Overalls. The Beverly Hillbillies Dieter will have several pairs: pinstripe for those meetings in the financial district; perhaps a tasteful paisley for Christopher Street or a little sortie to the Morton Street pier; simple navy blue for the easternmost of the Hamptons or a Bel Air luncheon. Basic black for those formal hoe-downs.

Polecat. A dinner guest who insists upon your sharing an order of tortellini to start.

Polk salad. One of the delicious leafy greens found in abundance in your garden. Closely resembles mustard greens or collard greens. Third cousin, once-removed, to spinach. Sister to turnip greens.

Southern champagne. Coca-Cola. It used to be the real thing; it still is. Always the best. Accept no substitutions.

Switch. A slender branch from a tree. Sometimes used by pa with great reluctance in spankings; also used by city heavies with considerably less reluctance to ward off muggers.

THE FRANKLY MEANT presents

THE BEVERLY HILLS DIET
KEEPSAKE COLLECTION

After you have seen how much *The Beverly Hillbillies Diet* can do for you, you will realize that food is more than any old group.

For the many of you who appreciate what the finest in Americana doodads can mean to your decor, the Frankly Meant is pleased to offer this limited edition of collectibles:

BRONZE OR COPPER
Baby's First Porkchops lovingly crafted to become lustrous bookends.

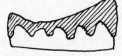

The Bride's First Cake
A priceless memento of your first married dessert.

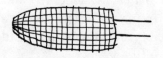

IN STERLING
Corn-on-the-Cob Skewers

The Beverly Hillbillies
Backyard Range Finder

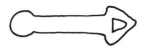

The Bottle Opener

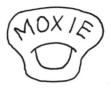

Grapette Cufflinks   *Okra Earrings*

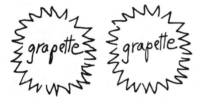   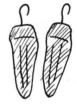

The Catfish Doorstop

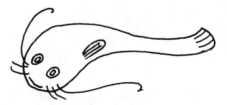

The Grits Keyring

10
Some Final Inspirational Words

Well, you did it.

After eating up a storm, you're back in shape and your dance card is filling up again. And, you no longer have to arrive at the cotillion or the Polo Lounge in a double-wide buckboard.

You gritted your teeth through a week of grits and you are looking positively grand.

You may have muttered a few unkind things about us while chewing your four hundredth mouthful of turnip greens, but now you're just a fiend for fatback.

And haven't you found that walking has got to be a habit with you?

No more compulsive city eating; Country Combining has become a natural fack.

You may have thought you couldn't last six weeks but you did, and now you couldn't last two days without our cast-iron cuisine.

Whatever your address, now you will always be a fit hillbilly—in touch with your body, easily able to touch your toes.

Neighbor, you are back to the basics. You are picking in tall cotton. And, as Phil Harris used to say, "That's what I like about the South."

Welcome to the World of the Golden Grit!